HEAD & NECK CANCER

CANCER

THE SECOND ENCOUNTER

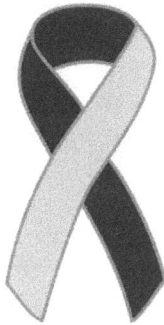

STEPHEN MCPHERSON

Published in Australia by Sid Harta Publishers Pty Ltd,
ABN: 34 632 585 203
17 Coleman Parade, GLEN WAVERLEY VIC 3150 Australia
Telephone: +61 3 9560 9920, Facsimile: +61 3 9545 1742
E-mail: author@sidharta.com.au

First published in Australia 2020
This edition published 2022
Copyright © Stephen McPherson 2020

Cover design, typesetting: WorkingType (www.workingtype.com.au)

Head and Neck Cancer — The Second Encounter
Stephen McPherson
ISBN: 978-1-925707-15-1
Ebook: 978-0-6455257-6-2
pp94

Dedication

This book is dedicated to a number of key people who are responsible for my survival with my latest encounter with head and neck cancer.

To ensure that this patient survived I wish to thank all of the medical practitioners who, without their skills and training, would not have successfully diagnosed and treated this condition.

To the people who actually kept me alive, the wonderful nurses at Ward 6A of Fiona Stanley Hospital, Murdoch Perth. Their dedication to their profession and patient care is a credit to each and every one of them.

One nurse in particular who I believe went above and beyond what was required for my survival, is the Surgical Head and Neck Coordinator Nurse in Clinic 5, Fiona Stanley Hospital. This wonderful lady provided this survivor with advice about the whole process and was there every step of the way. Her job is to take care of the patient by addressing any issues, concerns, questions and problems that they may have, not only prior to the surgery but also afterwards and for the next five years.

This made the whole process a little more comfortable, knowing that there was professional support for me at all times.

The final person that this book is dedicated to is the most important lady in my life, my wife Abigail. Without her constant support and encouragement, this survivor questions whether it would have been all possible.

Thank you to all of you from my heart.

Stephen McPherson

About the author

Stephen Mcpherson comes from Mandurah in Western Australia. Stephen spent the last twenty-five years performing Occupational Safety and Health roles for various companies in Australia. Stephen started his own consultancy and built it up to include clients from all over the world.

In 2016, Stephen started studying full-time doing law at Notre Dame University in Fremantle Perth. He had about twelve months to go to finish his degree, wanting to specialise in Safety, Workers Compensation and Industrial Relations.

Before undertaking a job in this field, Stephen spent ten years in the Royal Australian Air Force as a Policeman, and this is where he gets most of his discipline, positivity and determination from.

Stephen is the oldest of two children and is currently living in Perth. As a result of the cancer, Stephen lost both his career, business and future as a lawyer.

One thing that was lacking in Western Australia when Stephen started this journey, was support from external agencies and he had to rely on family.

So, Stephen started the Perth Head and Neck Cancer Support Group and a head and neck cancer charity called the Western Australian Head and Neck Cancer Support Foundation.

WARNING: Some photographs in this book may be confronting and upsetting. Please use caution. They are designed so that patients will have an idea on what to expect and will not be alarmed when waking up or seeing what they look like. You just won't be as ugly as the author.

CONTENTS

THE FIRST ENCOUNTER

My first encounter with head and neck cancer occurred in July 2015. As a typical Australian bloke, I never was very keen on going to the doctor, I had a 'she'll be alright attitude,' especially if it involved going to a specialist. In February 2015, I had an obstruction in my nose. I got a referral to Murdoch ENT Clinic at the Wexford Centre Murdoch Perth, Western Australia.

I did not do anything about it until I made and attended an appointment in June 2015. While there, I asked the doctor to look at three little grey growths that were sitting on the side of my tongue, which had come up the week before.

He said, 'Yeah we can have a look at that for you. I have to knock you out to remove the polyp in the nose, so I will take some biopsies of these growths and see what they are.'

The following week, I was in hospital, not knowing I was getting my first head and neck cancer operation. The biopsies were done, and the tests would be back in a couple of days. I went home the next day after the operation.

Now you know it is not good when a doctor's office rings you two days after the biopsy saying the doctor wants to see you now! Your heart sinks knowing that he is not inviting you to his office to let you know you are good looking or for a coffee.

I went to his office. The doctor's pleasantries were what you expect. 'Get on with it and give me the bad news,' I say. 'The biopsies showed that you have three growths of Squamous Cell Carcinoma. This is an aggressive type of cancer. The best course of action is to cut it out. I can do it tomorrow,' he says. 'No, I need a couple of days to get some affairs in order,' I said. The date for my first operation was Wednesday 1st July 2015.

Some background history about me. I have never smoked and didn't drink alcohol. I ate relatively healthy and on occasions did some exercise. So how did I get Squamous Cell Carcinoma of the tongue?

I did a lot of research and spoke to my GP doctor at Port Kennedy Medical Centre in Perth, who just happened to be the Australian Medical Association President for Western Australian at the time. He advised me that the

Australian Medical Association had seen an increase in the number of males, especially around my age that have this type of cancer.

It comes from the Human Papillomavirus (HPV). Isn't this the thing that causes cancer in female cervix? 'Yes.' Nothing more to be said about how I got it in my tongue.

In 2010, the government ran a campaign to inoculate 12-year-old girls against HPV. However, at the time nothing was done for males and no advice was issued for males of any age on the dangers of contracting HPV through oral sex. Being sexually active since 1975, I could have contracted it at any time and it just lay dormant, until now.

The next Wednesday I had the operation. The ENT surgeon cut out the growths. When I was in my room, I was visited by the doctor and he advised on what he had done. 'Great,' I said. 'All gone.'

I was at home recovering, and you guessed it, I got another call from the ENT Clinic saying that the specialist wanted to see me again. I go and see him and he advises me that while the operation was successful, the safety margin was of the smallest margins and he would like to go back in and cut out some more of my tongue out. 'How much are you going to take?' said I. 'In total one third of your tongue. This provides for a greater safety margin.'

Now with stiches in the tongue, talking, eating and drinking were a little hard. Boy, knowing what I do now I wish I had the same problem where I could still talk and eat.

Second operation on my tongue was completed and I am now cancer free, with better safety margins. Now it's a case of monthly, quarterly and then six-month check-ups over the next five years and annual PET Scans.

I continue life as normal, as the operation did not impact on eating, drinking or talking.

THE SECOND ENCOUNTER

In November 2017, I had my last quarterly check-up and was advised to now make them six monthly instead. By now, things were going really well with PET Scans and the regular examinations, both showed no return of the cancer.

In January 2018, I had to have an MRI on my head and neck for shoulder pain that I was having at the time.

I mention this, as the MRI showed no indications of cancer or any other growth activity, from my shoulders up.

My first six monthly check-up took place on the 25th of May 2018. The specialist said, 'I don't know if you have noticed or not, but your tongue is swollen.' The swelling had come up in the space of four months to the stage where it could be visually observed by the specialist. As I was due for my annual PET scan, it was undertaken to ascertain if there was any indication of cancer or anything else.

The results indicated that there were a number of hot spots on my tongue, including the muscles in the base of the tongue this time. Not a good sign. The specialist said, 'Let's take a biopsy to ascertain what it is.' Next week I had three biopsies on my tongue taken.

The following week I had an appointment with the specialist and was told that, 'the biopsies showed both cancerous and pre-cancerous cells. Let's do an MRI to see what we are actually dealing with.' An MRI was undertaken, and a follow-up appointment made.

The following week, I had the next appointment with my specialist where he advised that they had a better idea of what they were dealing with and wanted to take another biopsy of my tongue.

A week later, I had a second set of biopsies of my tongue taken. The day after the biopsies, I went home and was advised that I would be contacted once the results came in.

Trying to talk, eat and drink is a lot harder with stiches in your tongue and while in pain.

I went to see the specialist the following week and he told

me the not-so-great news. 'Stephen sorry but your cancer has returned and with a vengeance this time, you are what we call a Stage Four cancer patient. The MRI indicates that at least 75% of your tongue has what appears to be cancer in it, including the muscles of the base of the tongue and the glands in the neck.'

For the last 33 years, I had only had medical treatment at private facilities. However, my specialists, while practising out of both public and private hospitals, suggested that I attend Fiona Stanley Hospital Murdoch Perth, being a public hospital in Western Australia.

The reason being is the Ear, Nose and Throat team, work as part of an integrated management team. For this reason, all of my treatment would be coordinated and monitored by all departments involved. He would still be my treating doctor and would oversee everything.

At the time I was very reluctant but accepted his suggestion. Now as you can imagine the feelings and emotions that start to rise are huge.

I started to think about what was going to happen to me. Would I survive this ordeal? Would I get the same care and treatment as what I do in private hospitals? Would I be able to speak again? What am I going to do for employment? Would I be able to eat again?

These thoughts kept on coming up. I would wake up in the middle of the night thinking about what was going to happen to me and if I would not only survive, but live a normal life. And if not, then what was I going to do? I lost many nights of sleep thinking about this.

These are just a few of the hundreds of questions that raced through my mind. It was normal to have these feelings, doubts and questions, so my psychologist told me.

I needed advice and guidance as to what to do. I had seen the same GP for the last twenty-five years, someone that I not only trusted but knew very well. I went to my GP and we spoke.

One thing that he told me, and I have never forgotten this is, 'that regardless of what or where they want to do something, accept it. The reason being is, what they are doing comes from true, tried and proven protocols that work. Start picking the ones you want or don't want and the whole treatment process will more than likely fall over. They are specialists and they know what they are doing.'

At this point, I was a safety consultant and full-time law student, with one year to finish my law degree, both of which require me to speak to clients. So, what happens if I cannot talk, what am I going to do for a living? How am I going to communicate with people in general or day to day?

The thoughts and doubts continued throughout this whole process.

I came to the conclusion that I had enough on my plate dealing with the diagnosis and what I was facing, and decided to **take it one day at a time**. I found that dealing with one thing at a time was the best approach.

Resolve the issue and move on, I told myself. Every so often, go back and make sure that the resolutions will still work with the new things you have found and put in place.

Now I want to point out something that I attribute my successful treatment and recovery to: it is support. The one thing that I found was a lack of support for patients with head and neck cancer from your normal cancer support agencies. There was a lot of support for a lot of other cancers but just not head and neck. This made what I was going through even harder.

Throughout the whole process, my wife was beside me at all meetings, appointments and tests and was my greatest support and still is today.

You are dealing with a lot of emotions and pressures that the last thing you want to do is miss something that is vital information that someone tells you, because you are concentrating on something someone else just said.

Take a notebook and write things down.

Having someone important in your life reduces the pressure and you have someone to talk to when things get bad.

And things were going to get bad. I never realised how a human can have so many different emotions at either the same time or in quick succession.

I expected it and was ready for it. That's how I dealt with the issue. I used humour and tried not to take things too seriously (don't get me wrong this was serious but I still kept my sense of humour). I always tried to find a funny or humorous side to what was happening.

For example, I didn't have to eat things I did not like. The cost of me eating was significantly reduced, as my feed was on a prescription and each prescription lasts about two and half weeks, with what I consume per meal.

This actually allowed me to handle the situation better. I learned not to get too worked up and let emotions take over. I learned to relax, see a situation from a more positive angle, and acknowledged that if things did get out of control, I would be able to let things go more easily and move on with my life.

A positive mindset helped me get through things.

FIONA STANLEY HOSPITAL

My first appointment was at ENT Clinic 5, Fiona Stanley Hospital. It started off with one doctor telling me what the process was going to be and then he informed me that I would meet the team in a minute.

The next thing, as if on cue, 18 people came into the room, the team. I had everyone from the head of ENT surgery, to the head of plastic surgery as well as their support doctors and nurses. There were also speech therapists and dietitians in the room.

This added to my stress and panic and I asked myself: 'Am I really that bad that I need this many doctors?'

They all introduced themselves. I wasn't listening to them because I was still getting over the number of people that came in and they all wanted to have a look at my tongue and feel my throat. Given it was now four weeks since my last CT and MRI scans, new update scans were organised.

They advised that the course of treatment was the removal of the affected area of my tongue. Indications were that this was going to be about 75% of the tongue including the base muscles.

After surgery I would undergo a course of chemoradiation therapy to ensure that any microscopic cancer cells are killed.

I asked what the survivability rate of this type of surgery was. 'There is no easy way to say this,' said the specialist. 'The operation survivability rate is 12%. Whereas, the survivability rate of this type of cancer after five years is 63%.' I knew that I was going to be both, the 12% and 63%, that was for sure.

EMOTIONS

Crap! I knew sex would kill me but not literally. Panic was the first thing that set in. What does it mean to lose 75% of my tongue?

I had a lot of questions and concerns and I could not think straight.

The following questions ran through my head: Will I be able to eat and drink? Would I be able to speak? If I cannot speak what am I going to do for a living? Do I continue with my law degree? Do I close my safety consultancy down? If I can't eat or drink how do I live? Will that be conducive to our lifestyle? Will I be able to go overseas on holidays or for that matter fly in general? With all the surgery, will I look the same. Will my wife still love me with all the scars? How am I going to live in general? How are people going to understand me if I cannot talk? Do I have to learn sign language, how do I do that?

These were just some of the hundred questions and concerns I had at the time. A lot of nights' sleep were lost worrying about what was happening to me. There were a lot of other ones which all were and are normal, so my psychologist told me.

It was all about me and the one thing that I forgot was my wife and what she must have been going through.

That evening we sat down and had a heart-to-heart discussion about our feelings, fears and concerns. She had concerns that I might have contracted the virus from her. The solution was to go and have the test and find out, but it didn't matter where I got it from, it was about dealing with the cards we were dealt with and making the most of it.

It helped both of us so much knowing what the other person was thinking and going through. Of course, it was very emotional but that was to be expected. All in all, we were and still are there for each other.

At the end we agreed that regardless of what came our way we should always talk to each other and express our true concerns and feelings on a regular basis and be true and honest about what we were thinking and worried about.

My wife had the HPV test and she was clear, which gave her great peace of mind, that it wasn't her that gave me this virus.

I started many hours on the internet researching what I could about this procedure called Sub Total Glossectomy, the medical name for the surgery that I was going to receive.

One website that was very helpful was **www.beyond5. org.au**. The website had a lot of information applicable to what I was about to undertake.

However, when researching you have to keep in mind that not all of the things you find out are going to be applicable to you and what you are going through. Keep an open mind and ask a lot of questions of your medical practitioners and most importantly make sure you get your questions answered, don't let them brush over the question but make sure you get the answer to satisfy your question and you understand the answer.

Now some doctors think they are superior (for which you cannot blame them, given the work they have done to get to where they are) but they need to realise that they are dealing with a person who is scared, ill and has a lot of emotions going through them. Make sure you get your questions answered and don't let the person off the hook until you do. You need to have your fears addressed and this was one of my biggest problems because I couldn't always understand the answers they were giving me.

How did I get the answers to the questions I had?

Fortunately, this is where the Head and Neck Coordinator Nurse came into her own. If I could not find an answer from any source, I would ask her, she would source the answer and get back to me in a very acceptable timeframe.

I think there were only a couple of questions she could not answer, and they were medical procedural questions. But my doctors answered them for me. I also asked many other questions when I saw both the Head and Neck Coordinator and the doctors and I wasn't afraid to ask the dumbest questions.

PLANNING FOR SURGERY

My research showed that as part of the surgery process they would insert a tracheostomy tube into my neck. This would allow the mouth to heal and of course allow me to breathe without any obstructions.

This would also mean that I would not be able to talk after surgery, for how long, no one knew. It was a matter of waiting and seeing, if ever again.

How could I communicate with the nurses and doctors to tell them how I am, or what I needed? I could use pen and paper, which would mean I could go through a lot of paper and if my handwriting was not the best, because of drugs, then what?

I found a website called **www.magicwhiteboard.com.au** (they are based in Perth and respond very quickly). They supply whiteboard notebooks. I purchased an A5 and A4 size notebook along with a few pens and cleaning materials. The advantage is the notebooks are reusable and you can wipe the pages clean. Okay, that is great, but what about if my handwriting was not the best?

I went to the Apple store and found two apps that convert text to speech. The first one was for free and is called **Text to Speech**. Good for basic communication, the only downside is it is a bit of a hassle saving commonly used phases.

The next app was **Predictable**. This one is not for free and it cost AUD$298.00. The advantage of this app was that it allowed the user to save commonly used phases, different languages, and male or female voices. It was a lot more user-friendly and adaptable to what one would want and need.

Communication with doctors, nurses, loved ones and visitors was solved.

I dealt with one problem at a time, but I knew that at some point I was going to feel down and sorry for myself. This was a dangerous situation and a fragile time as depression can lead to all sort of problems and add complications to the recovery and healing processes. I needed to avoid this as much as possible, while also allowing myself to feel sorry for myself from time to time.

How did I keep a positive attitude to what I was going

through? The biggest problem I anticipated was the number of times that I would be depressed and ask basic questions like: 'Why me?' or 'What is going to happen to me?' 'Am I going to survive?' 'How am I going to come out of this?'

This is normal and acceptable, but I could not focus on that. I was going to spend a lot of time by myself and if I started to get depressed it would be difficult to come back from it.

While I had a positive attitude, I needed to improve and ensure that it remained. I designed five A4 posters that had simple words on them like 'I'm in the fight of my life and I'm going to win.' 'I'm in the fight of my life and I will win.' 'I will NOT give up.' 'Strength, Courage, Faith and Hope.' and 'Losing is NOT an Option.' Simple messages, but something that would keep me positive.

I printed the five out and took them to the hospital with me. When I got to the ward I asked if they could put them up around the room and they said not a problem. Wherever I looked in my room, there was one of these posters. They kept me positive and focused by not letting me feel sorry for myself.

Don't get me wrong, there were and are going to be times when you will feel sorry for yourself, I did. I often thought about the big question 'why me' along with a few hundred more. That's fine allowing you to feel sorry for yourself for a couple of minutes but you have to get back to staying positive and focusing on recovery.

A positive mind and attitude **does** go a long way to aid recovery and healing.

Planning what you are going to need and how you are going to do it before you go into hospital, is much better than trying to do it once you have had the operation and are not able to move, talk or communicate.

If nothing else, it will keep you focused on something other than what you are about to undergo. It also makes your life easier once in hospital because you have the tools that you need to help you deal with everyday problems which you will face.

One of the biggest things that I found was the fact that technology is ever-changing and can be relied upon to do many more things. Who knows what is to come in the future. Some of the text-to-speech applications allow for you to use your own voice.

Get in front of a video camera or as I did, my laptop camera, and make a video of a very long message to your loved one.

A couple of reasons: if for whatever reason you do not

survive the operation, you can tell your loved one what you are feeling, your relationship and any other personal message you want to leave them. This gives them something positive to remember you by.

Then record your life. Start where you were born and all the things you can remember about growing up. Include both the high and low moments. This will become your voice bank. If you want to use the text-to-speech application to use your voice you have a very detailed bank of voice information to enable that to happen, such as various tones, pitches and sounds.

FINAL CHECK UP

So, I had another appointment to get the results of the latest MRI and CT scans. Six doctors entered the room. This was not good, I just knew it, just as nothing was in these moments. Since the last scan it appeared that I was now looking at closer to 90% of my tongue being removed due to cancer, this also included the base muscles and some glands in my neck as well.

I questioned what would happen if I didn't have the surgery. The head surgeon said, 'Then you have had your last Christmas because you will not be here for the 2018 Christmas.' Four and half months, great. 'Okay let's do it, I will have to learn to deal with the results and/or side effects,' I said.

The doctors then explained the process. They would first cut my neck and insert a tracheostomy tube, then cut from my lip, down my chin, to just above the tracheostomy tube and then from ear to ear. They would then remove the jawbone and start cutting out the cancer.

Once the cancer has been removed, the ENT team would then hand over to the plastics team.

The plastics team started to tell me what they were going to do. First, they would cut out a piece of my right thigh muscle and place it into the area where the tongue was. This would be stitched down and I would not be able to move. This was to protect the mouth floor.

SURGICAL PROCESS

Feeding Tube

The team at ENT Clinic 5 advised that I would get a feeding tube (Percutaneous Endoscopic Gastrostomy - PEG) inserted prior to the surgery.

This way it would allow me the opportunity to learn how to use it and get comfortable with it prior to the main surgery. The two options were nasal tube or stomach tube.

Because I cannot stand anything in the back of my throat (bad gag reflex), I opted for a feeding tube directly out of my stomach. This would also reduce the potential for people to stare at me, as they do when they see something different. After all, this was more than likely going to be long-term if not permanent, particularly in my case.

I was glad that I took the tube through my stomach option, as when I woke up from the main surgery, I discovered that I could not talk, eat or swallow.

The pain was very high. The feeding tube was normal to me and I was not worried about having food, medicine or water, as it was now second nature.

Before you go into hospital for the main operation, I urge you to go out for a meal. Make it your favourite meal and treat it as the last meal you are going to ever eat. Mine was steak with garlic prawns with lots of vegetables, followed by apple pie and ice cream and Earl Grey tea. I can still taste it.

The reason for this is that you do not know if you are going to be able to eat normally again. This will give you something to work towards after the operation.

Ideally have the meal with your loved one or family. Make them part of your journey and experience, not just in this moment, but through the complete journey. Their support is of utmost importance to your survivability; I honestly believe that.

My wife was with me throughout the whole experience and as she said I went through the physical side, she the emotional side, which I think is worse. My mother-in-law (who I get on with) contacted me or came to see me every day to check on me, and even now. I told her to make it once a week, as it was not necessary because I am doing so much better now.

THE DAY

Well the day, 1ˢᵗ August 2018, that I had been worried about arrived. I made my way to Fiona Stanley Hospital for 6 a.m. A nice bright early start. All the hospital legal paperwork was done and signed, as well as my consent for the surgery to take place.

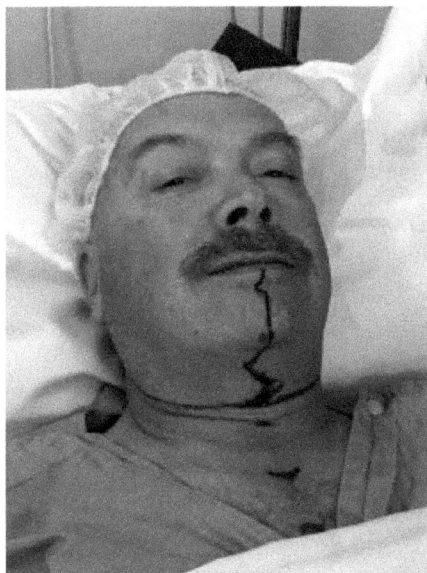

I said my goodbyes to my wife, who was still by my side. I was taken into the surgical theatre to meet the surgeons who went through the surgery process. I was given a needle and told 'goodnight Stephen.' That was the last I knew about the process, at that time.

Intensive Care Unit

Well I woke up, that was a bonus, in the Intensive Care Unit. I was one of the 12% that survived the operation. The first person I recall seeing was, you guessed it, my wife. The nurses tell me where I am and the fact that being in ICU means I have one nurse to look after me twenty-four hours per day while I am here, which will be for a few days. One of the surgeons came in and explained the process to me.

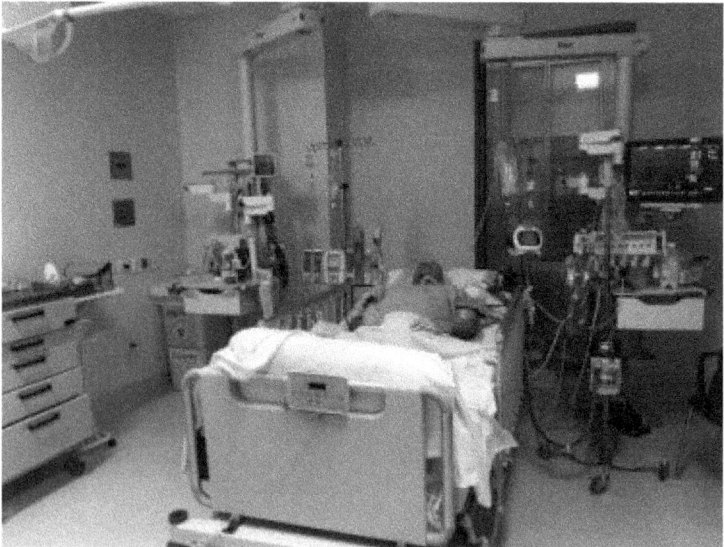

ENT Operation

I was on the operating table for 16 hours. The Ear, Nose and Throat team started the operation with the insertion of the tracheostomy tube, then an incision through my lip and a cut through my jaw, then down to my neck.

The cut around my neck, from ear to ear, had removed my jawbone to make room for the operation.

My tongue was then removed piece by piece. Each piece was examined for cancerous cells before removing the next piece. They finally stopped with approximately the removal of 88% of my tongue and all my base muscles before no more cancerous cells were in the tissues. They took approximately another 2% as a safety margin. In total 90% of my tongue was gone, that's for sure.

They started to remove glands from my neck. They removed 50 glands from each side before they were 100% happy that there were no cancerous cells in the glands. Well that left 100 on either side. This took 10 hours.

Plastics Operation

The Plastics team then took over the surgery for another 6 hours and did what they said they were going to do. They cut a section of my right thigh muscle out and used it to fill in the tongue space. It was sewn in place and could not move.

The incision was 23 centimetres long and 10 centimetres wide and about 5 centimetres deep. I just wished that they shaved the leg before they cut the piece out. I would include a picture that we took, but it is not pretty. I'm sure you get the idea.

Later what I found out was that I had hairs on my mouth flap, and it tickled the roof of my mouth, most annoying.

The final result of the surgery was:

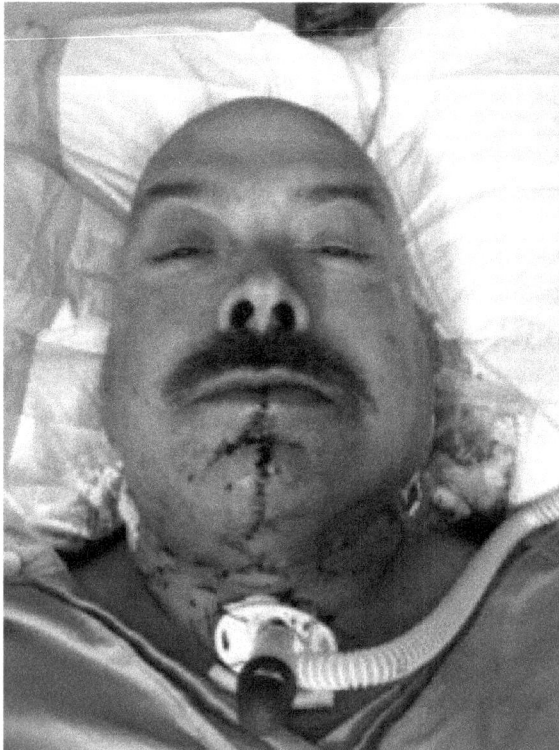

I asked, 'So what are the plastic bags I have sticking out of my head on either side.' The doctor replied, 'they are drains to allow excess fluid to drain out of the wound. You also have one on the leg as well.'

Well the stay in ICU was relatively uneventful. The only thing I put in place was the restriction that only my wife was allowed to visit me in the ICU.

I needed time to recover and get used to how I looked and not being able to talk before entertaining visitors. Remember it is about you and what you want. The surgery took a toll on both my body and mind.

RECOVERY

Ward 6A

After a couple of days in ICU, I was transferred to Ward 6A of Fiona Stanley Hospital. The nurses were very caring, understanding and professional in patient care and they always explained everything I needed to know, throughout the duration of my whole stay there.

Because I had a tracheostomy, I had to be in a room close to the nurses' station. This was reassuring as if anything did go wrong, they were close by.

For the first couple of days I was fed through an intravenous drip. But then they had to start to feed me through a PEG tube. Now this was where I started to have a few problems.

I am not only a type two diabetic, but I also have Crohn's

Disease. Crohn's Disease is the narrowing of the bowel and in my case is treated by tablets.

The problem is the tablets cannot be crushed and put through the PEG and I cannot swallow them, because I had no tongue and my mouth was swollen.

So, when I started to be fed via my PEG, it exacerbated my Crohns and I had up to eighteen or twenty bowel motions a day. I do use the term bowel motions loosely, because they did not resemble anything I know as bowel motions. In fact, other than not being yellow, it reminded me of my kids' nappies.

The nurses were concerned and spoke to the dietitian. They wanted the dietitian to change my food, so they changed it. It worked for a time, while in hospital and it certainly reduced the number of bowel motions.

The doctors and nurses got used to me using my app to talk and it became very normal for both of us.

For distant family not so much, as there were times when they did not understand that I had to use an app to talk. But we got there and eventually we were able to have conversations.

That's how you know who your friends are by who comes to see you in hospital. Needless to say, our friends just all disappeared and none of them came to see me in hospital. But saying that, through the power of social media, I put on my Facebook page that I was in hospital and what happened was that some very old (and when I say old I mean long term not age-wise) friends came to see me. I had not seen some of them for thirty odd years.

I still see one of them, even today, and it is great to have a friend who I grew up with and get along with, after all this time.

Infection

It was a week and a half after the operation and I started to feel very sore and red around the neck, as the below picture shows.

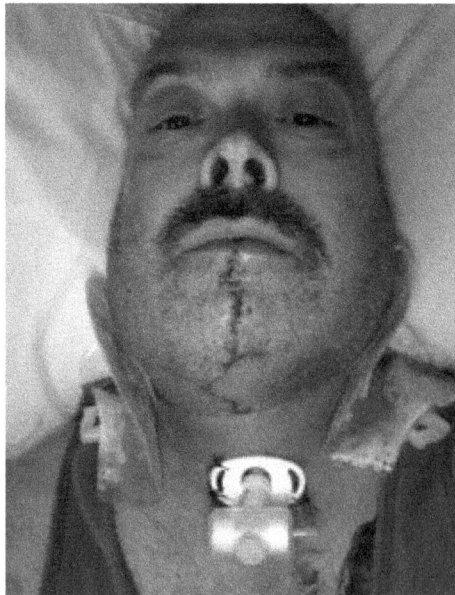

Congratulations Stephen, you have a wound infection and we will have to go back in and clean it out. One must remember that while all care is taken to ensure hospitals are clean and sterile, sometimes things do still happen.

That's all right, it was a slight setback in my recovery. The doctor explained the process and I was happy to sign the consent form.

Another surgery; they opened up my neck and scrubbed the wound clean and stitched me back up. I woke up back in my room on Ward 6A.

No infection anymore. It was again time to focus on recovering from what had happened.

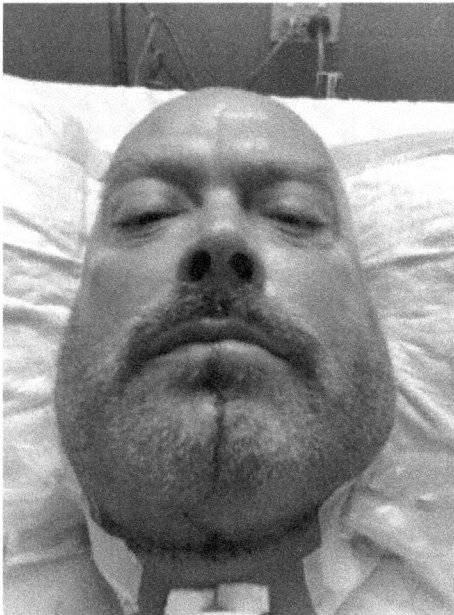

After this latest surgery I did have a couple of hiccups. Twice I had code blue incidents. Code blue is where a patient has airway problems and the ward staff needs urgent assistance.

Boy I was worried when I was struggling to breathe but believe me, not as worried as I was when 21 staff members crashed into my room. Doctors, Nurses, Specialists, I had them all.

Ten minutes later, the matter was resolved, and I was breathing relatively normally and my oxygen levels were slowly coming back up.

When it happened the second time, I was expecting the number of staff members and was not disappointed. I have to say the response to an emergency like this was one of the best that I had ever seen.

Unfortunately, in my life I have dealt with numerous emergencies and have been to hospitals all over the world for one reason or another and not always for me. The response time and the professional people who attended to me were very impressive and reassuring.

PROGRESS

So, time was ticking. Three weeks and I was having more positive moments than negative moments, but the key was that I was getting better.

Allow yourself to have those negative moments but don't focus or let them consume you. However, what happened next was so funny.

Smurf Test

Now, we all know that Smurfs are blue, so you can imagine what I was thinking when the doctors told me that they are going to do a Smurf test on me. 'A what? I have to see how many Smurfs I can see?' Remember I was on great pain killers and I didn't have to worry about constipation side effects.

The doctor explained that this was where they place blue dye into your mouth to see if there are any leaks. From the blue dye they would be able to ensure that your mouth was sealed, and if things were where they were supposed to be.

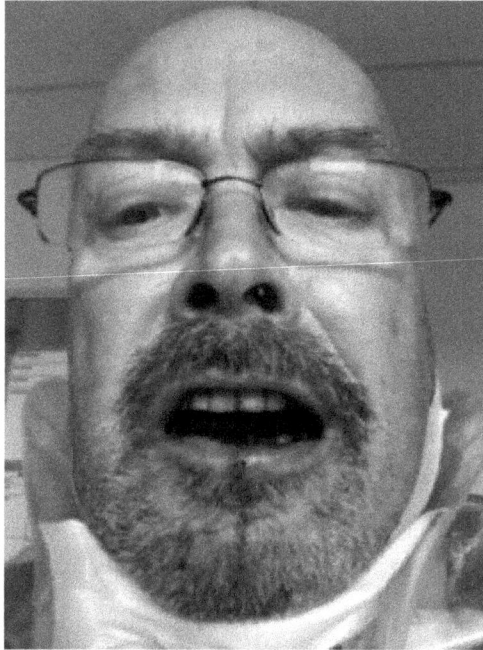

Smurf test undertaken and passed, no leaks, thank you surgeons. But let me tell you, the blue dye takes some time before is disappears and it's funny when visitors come and see you, looking all worried.

Now remember I told you about my sense of humour? Well let me tell you that I had fun with the dye. I told visitors various things like that it was a disease that I had contracted, that my flap was dying, that I tried putting lipstick on and missed or that I got hungry and ate a nurse's lipstick ... all sorts of things. But boy, it sure looked like I ate some Smurfs that's for sure!

Progress Continuing

So, things were going well, and I was getting better as each day passed by. I had physios coming around to take me for daily walks, dietitians checking on me, nurses constantly monitoring me and doctors checking to make sure that I was going in the right direction and that there were no problems.

It did take time and I was under no illusion that it was only going to be a week's visit. In the end it was just short of five weeks.

After the Smurf test, I had the tracheostomy tube capped for a while, before the decision was made for it to be removed. I had no airway problems and was breathing on my own and had been for a while. A doctor and nurse came in, set up the table and removed the tube, a two-minute job.

The result a hole in my neck.

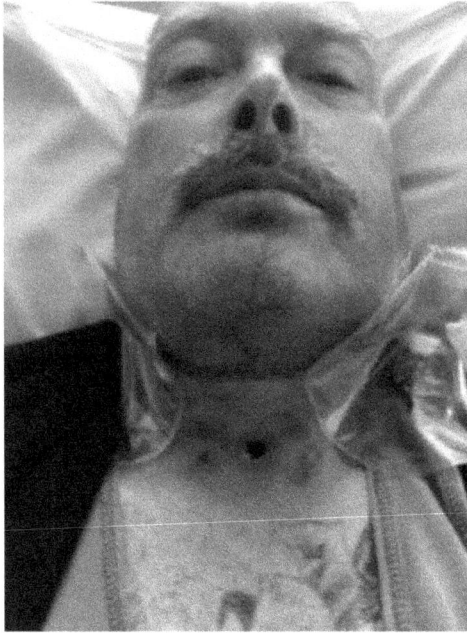

This was dressed with a special bandage and dressing. The important part was that they placed a heart monitor dot on the dressing. EVERY time you spoke, you had to place a finger on the dot so that you could allow the wound to heal and stop air from escaping.

The more times you do this, the quicker the wound will heal, and it is safer for you.

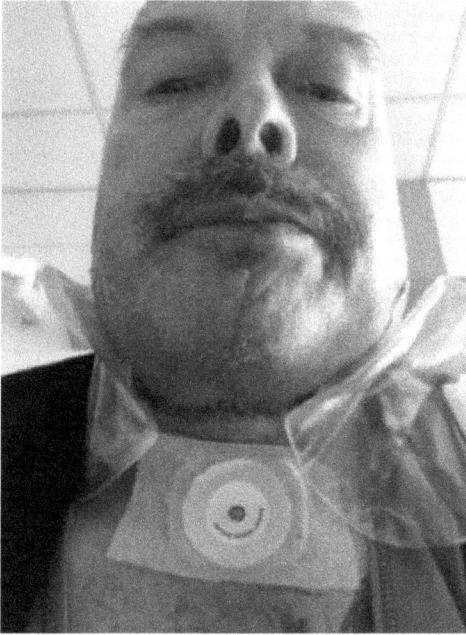

During the same week the two drains in my neck stopped draining fluids into the bags. After a couple of days with nothing, the decision was made to remove the drains from both my neck and leg. As you can see from the photo below these were not small drains and I was amazed at how long they were.

What you can see on the outside was just as long on the inside. Unfortunately, I was not able to get photos of them being removed but did manage once to get photos when the bags were being changed.

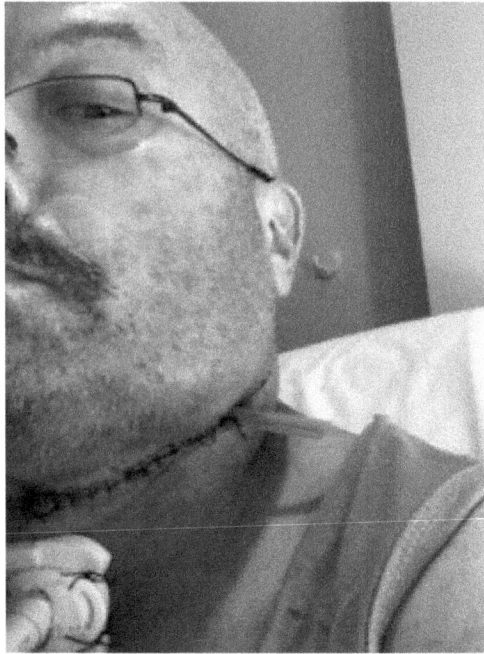

Things were progressing well, eventually. Discussions actually got around to me going home. While very keen to go home, I did not want to rush it, after all, I had just undergone two major operations and needed to get my head ready for my next step.

Discharge

The day came, goodbye Fiona Stanley Hospital Ward 6A. I was discharged and taken home by my lovely wife. Now let me tell you something, not only did I lose weight but I also had a lack of energy and stamina.

DON'T overdo it. Listen to the person caring for you and follow all the instructions given to you at the hospital. I know several times it was a struggle just to go to the lounge room or more importantly the toilet. I tired so quickly and had numerous senior naps on the lounge suite.

The plan was to have four weeks recovery at home taking it **easy**. Then an appointment would be organised for me to attend radiation therapy, in my case at Genesis Cancer Care at Fiona Stanley Hospital.

RADIATION THERAPY

Five weeks after discharge, I had my first appointment with the Genesis Cancer Care. Wonderful people and so professional and caring. One of the nurses took me into a room and explained to me in detail what was going to happen as she gave me a check-up.

First, they made a mask of my face. I lay on a table as a warm plastic sheet, with holes, was placed on my face and clamped to the table. This was then moulded to the shape of my face.

This was so that when I was having radiation treatment, they could shoot the radiation into the same correct spot every time.

I had a few problems as I was not comfortable being clamped to a table while not being able to move as they moulded the mask. I got over it and it was completed.

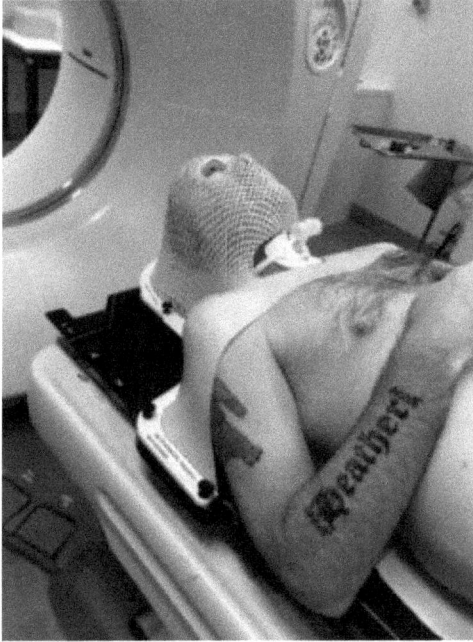

Then I had an appointment with a doctor who explained the radiation process for head and neck cancer and the side effects. The unfortunate part, as I was to discover later, was that not all the side effects were explained, even in the booklet they gave me.

I had to have radiation treatment five days a week: Monday — Friday for six weeks minimum and it would take me up to eighteen to twenty-four months to recover from both the operation and radiation therapy.

I didn't think it would be a short process or recovery time and I had to reassure myself and learn to have patience.

Treatment

In my work life I did many things. One of those was being a mines rescue paramedic and I was very comfortable being in small cramped spaces or even being trapped from time to time, so what happened next was and is so out of character for me.

I was in the radiation machine for the first time and they clamped my head to the table. I panicked, I had never suffered from claustrophobia, ever in my life.

The nurses worked extremely quickly to get the mask off me, and I sat up.

As you can see from the above photograph, this mask had hundreds of holes through it, so not only can you see but you could also breathe.

It took me five appointments (and the staff were very understanding and cooperative) before I could have the first radiation treatment and the only way I could do it was by playing my MP4 player with music in the background and concentrating on that and not the machine.

The cooking machine as I called it, or radiation machine, is awesome. First the table height is adjustable and rotates three hundred and sixty degrees. The arm that zaps you also rotates three hundred and sixty degrees.

The marks on the mask line up with the tattoos the nurses have put on me so that every time I am strapped on the table, the radiation is exactly where they want it. It is then checked with laser beams and if I am out of position the machine will not operate.

The treatment was not long. In my case it was about five or so minutes from start to finish and it went for seven and a half weeks.

Each time I had treatment it seemed to drain me of more energy and it was certainly uncomfortable afterwards. I felt burnt around the neck and lower jaw.

I know that I did not have to shave that part of my face because it was painful, but the other reason was that there was no hair there. The radiation burnt the hair follicles and killed most of them. Even now I still have a bald patch on my chin.

Emergency Problem

After ten sessions of radiation treatment I was at home and suddenly, I started to have problems breathing. When I say problems, I mean I was very short of breath and turning blue kinds of problems. My wife called an ambulance and administered first aid while waiting. I was rushed to Fiona Stanley Hospital with an airway occlusion. In other words, the radiation had burnt my airway and it was closing up. It was a side effect and it can happen, but no one told us, and it was not noted as a side effect in the booklet.

The treatment: Back to Ward 6A. 'Hello ladies I'm back.' I was laid on a bed and a tracheostomy tube was inserted but this time while I was awake, that was different.

This time I knew all about tracheostomy tube maintenance and use, so it was not as concerning as before. One week later I was discharged with a tube in my throat.

This stayed in place for the next five and a half months, well after treatment finished.

The tracheostomy tube was removed by, you guessed it, a nurse on Ward 6A, and afterwards I had a nice night's stay to make sure everything was okay and that I could survive without it. I was discharged the next day without any problems.

Radiation Continues

I had no other issues during my radiation treatment and was constantly monitored by both the doctors and nurses.

If you had an issue, you could front up to the nurses' counter and they would take care of you, very quickly and professionally.

At the end of the radiation therapy, the doctor told me the plan about moving forward. In my case, they wanted to do a PET Scan to ensure that they got all the cancer out. After that they would see me again in three months.

Lymphedema

The only other problem that I had was Lymphedema, this is where the fluids that would normally flow into the glands would go. But I had 50 removed from either side, so my face and neck blew up with excessive fluid. This was something that no one told me about before.

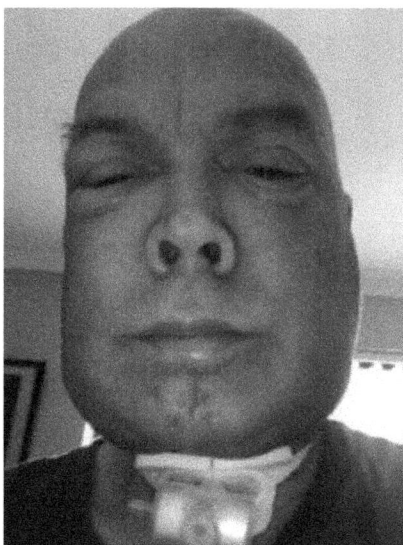

I attended a Lymphedema physio specialist at Fiona Stanley Hospital every fortnight and it was very successful.

After another four months, the Lymphadema should no longer be a problem anymore, as the fluids found a constant path to travel to the remaining glands.

PET Scan

The first PET Scan I had was a disaster, as for some reason, I panicked being in the machine. Now you have to remember that I have had five or six PET Scans before this one and didn't have a problem.

The operation certainly played with my mind.

Two months later I had another attempt at the PET Scan and a successful scan completed. This time I was inserted feet first, allowing my head more space.

Two weeks later I saw my specialist at the Wexford Centre and got the results. The words that we only dreamed about and wished for were: 'You are cancer-free, the operation and radiation were a success.'

Now I had another four and half years before I was deemed in remission.

Five years is the target and I know that I am going to be one of the 63% that survive this cancer. I know this for sure.

DEPRESSION

Right from the beginning while in the ICU, I contemplated what was going to happen to me, what I was going to do and I got depressed.

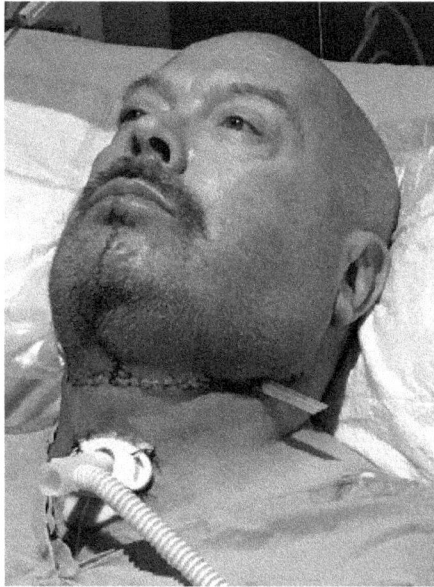

There were and still are times that I felt depressed, especially when I was alone not only in hospital, but more so when I was at home.

It was at this time, my wife took some time off when I came home from hospital. We both knew that could only last for so long as one of us had to bring in an income.

One day, I was sitting there feeling sorry for myself when all of a sudden, I had a mind shift. Instead of thinking how much I still had to do or how much I had lost, I started to realise how much I'd achieved. I am one of the 12% of people who survive the operation.

From that point on, I've always chosen to focus on the positives and especially on how much I've achieved in the past and how much confidence I can gain from all my past wins.

This gives me the belief and confidence that I can achieve any other task I set myself while staying motivated, persistent and committed to completing those tasks.

Sometimes you'll make that mindset shift yourself and sometimes you just need a kick in the arse from a loved one or good mate to remind you.

Mindset is a choice. Choose a positive one.

PAIN — Some words of advice

Don't be a hero; there is going to be pain and discomfort, accept it.

There are two ways to deal with it, painkillers and mindset.

Remember that everything will come to an end at some time.

I used my painkillers first thing in the morning and last thing at night, where I could. That way I did get a reasonable night's sleep.

During the day, I used my positive mindset and breathing exercises. Breathing can help you through some tough situations.

The tactical breathing method was deep, rhythmic,

belly breathing and it worked for me. Concentrating on the actual inhale and exhale of the breath will help you focus, relieve stress and help you cope by providing the body with a constant supply of oxygen.

Sometimes situations aren't ideal, and you can only do the best with what you have. You weigh it up, calculate the risks and make a decision based on the information and situation at hand. If you need painkillers take them, don't be a hero.

Just remember shitty situations always come to an end. As much as it sucks at the time, time itself will continue without fail and the suboptimal period you may find yourself in, will eventually dissipate.

EIGHT MONTHS ON

At this point I was eight months on from surgery, boy time flew by so quickly. The biggest thing for me was the removal of my tracheostomy tube and the difference it made to my life was incredible. Being able to have a shower whenever you wanted and to not have to worry about having someone there to change the dressings for you, and not having to wear a shower protector was great.

Some changes that I made to my rehabilitation treatment which took some pressure off the public health system was that I engaged my own speech therapist and dietitian.

This was to enable more frequent appointments and detailed rehabilitation specific to me.

Speech Therapy

The Speech Therapist I worked with works for herself out of the Wexford Centre in Murdoch and she was very good and highly recommended.

I can now hold a conversation, although I'm not always fully understood. I have been told by three speech therapists, a surgeon and a specialist that I am not supposed to be able to speak with 10% of a tongue.

Well if there was a way, I was certain that I would find it and that I would do it. A secret my therapist said to me was to use my lips instead of my tongue to accentuate and punctuate the words. It took some practice but is doable. Another piece of advice she offered was to slow down on speaking and take the time to pronounce the words correctly.

After the surgery, I was very limited on how far I could open my mouth and still am. My speech therapist has just got me a device called a TheraBite, which is designed for you to be able to open your mouth all the way over time by stretching and strengthening your muscles to go back into place. In one week, I made a progress of eight-millimetres.

Don't get me wrong I do have a speech impairment, and

some would say it is severe, but the only time I have to use my app these days is when I use the telephone.

For some reason, when I speak on the phone I am not understood. So, I use my Predictable app or the National Relay Service, problem solved.

I still have some saliva problems when I speak due to a build-up which restricts my speech. I find that if I drink water, I can usually cough it up. Otherwise it is a case of having something hot to drink and hopefully swallow it.

Also, when I wake up in the morning, I have a dry mouth and when I say dry, I mean really dry. Nothing that cannot be fixed with a drink of water, cup of coffee or tea.

At this point, the biggest thing that I have had to deal with is meals. I would sit there syringing liquid into my stomach while my family ate food.

After eight months I came to conquer this, by cooking for my family from time to time. Sure, I could not taste it, but I knew that I prepared it and could still smell it.

I also started to taste things, as much as I could. I started with sauces from meals then eventually I had chicken soup and vegetables. Now that sounds quite extraordinary, but I have to tell you it was puréed.

I could not use a spoon, so I put it in a cup and drank it. There is always a way, you just have to find a way around it.

I'm was able to have cups of tea, in my case, drink as much water as I wanted as well as fruit juice.

At this point, I had the confidence to try other things, but not without first discussing them with both my Speech Therapist and Dietitian. I didn't take any risks. I had come this far and didn't want to make a silly mistake by being overconfident.

DIETITIAN

My dietitian is a renowned elite sportsperson who holds several international marathon records. He is accredited as both a dietitian and a sports dietitian. He came to me highly recommended given my latest endeavour. I'll talk more about this later in the epilogue.

My dietitian went through everything that I was allowed to eat and drink. I had to maintain two litres of drink orally each day. I had to also make up my own thick shakes and have them from time to time. This ensured that I worked my throat muscles.

My dietitian has sourced a new feed (Elemental 028 extra) and I was now on 12 tetra packs of this special formula, along with protein, fibre and iron supplements. Progress will surprise.

I was still having some negative days and I sometimes wondered my worth, not only to my wife but to myself and my life. What was I going to do with myself day in and day out?

Was I to sit here every day surfing the internet and watching television?

Work would not be likely as my speech impairment was too severe, especially as it would be difficult to work as a lawyer or safety consultant.

Then I reminded myself that I was only eight months post-surgery and five months post-radiation. No rush, something will come along at the right time, I told myself, maybe it will be something that I have never considered before. If nothing came along, I would figure something out I was sure.

This picture is of me seven months post-surgery.

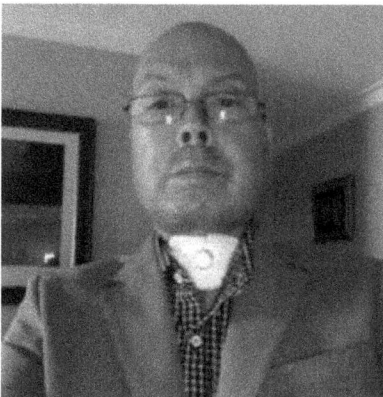

EPILOGUE

So, what does life look like for me after 18 months post operation and 14 months post-radiation? Still damn ugly, never mind, surgery doesn't fix everything!

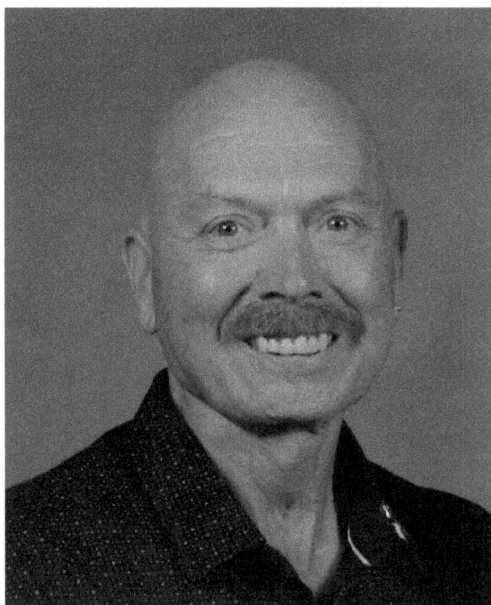

Well health-wise I have had no other major issues since radiation, or regarding what took place with the head and neck cancer operation.

Diet

My weight is now 75.2 kilograms up from the 67.1 kilograms which was when I was at my lightest. But still, a far way off the 110 kilograms I weighed prior to surgery.

I am happy with 75 kilograms and it is easy to stay at that weight. I just have to reduce the number of tetra packs I have per meal.

At this point, my dietitian still has me on four tetra packs of Elemental 028, two scoops of protein, a teaspoon and a half of fibre powder per meal. In addition, at breakfast I have 10 millilitres of iron supplements. And my blood work is in the middle of the normal levels.

Saliva Issues

These days, I still have saliva problems and on two occasions I have choked and collapsed on the ground not being able to breathe. Fortunately, each time I fell face-down and the obstacle that I choked on has dribbled out of my mouth.

On three other occasions I had choking episodes where I got down on all fours and was ready to collapse, but fortunately I managed to cough up the obstruction.

The problem is that the saliva is thick and it can be clear, green or even brown in colour, and given no tongue, it is not easy to move and/or swallow. Hot water helps.

Speech

I have been seeing my speech therapist since March 2019. My speech impairment is still what the majority of people would classify as severe and it is not going to get any better, no matter how often I see my speech therapist or how many exercises I do.

There is no need to see her as often these days and we agreed to make the appointments every three months, unless there is an issue.

It turns out my transplant shrunk more than expected and this resulted in me having the swallowing and choking problems that I am still having and the deterioration of my speech.

I resolved this by learning Auslan (Australian Sign Language) in an attempt to maintain my communication skills. I also noticed that I am using my phone app a little bit more often.

There have been two occasions where I have been verbally abused by people who I do not know. The insinuation was that I had a mental problem because of the way I spoke.

Psychological Issues

Now let me tell you about one of the incidents that happened to me about six months ago. I was at the shops buying a lotto ticket and the newsagent and I have a way of communicating that we can both understand. When I said goodbye, out of the corner of my eye I saw a lady standing there.

Unbeknown to me, she followed me out of the shops into the carpark. When I opened the car she started to yell at me questioning my ability to drive, asking if I had a drivers licence given I was a spastic (her words not mine and I do not for any reason condone the use of this word). She asked how could I have a drivers licence and threatened that she was going to call the police if I started the vehicle. I told her if she did not get out of my face, I would call the police for assault. She carried on and I drove off and left her there yelling at herself.

At the time I did not give it any thought, but later it started to shake me up and as it turned out, it really screwed me psychologically.

So, time went by and I was getting over the first incident of abuse and it was just before Christmas 2019. I had another run-in with a retail attendant who worked for a National Retail company, and who after a discussion yelled out, 'Are you just bloody stupid or just don't understand English'.

This time I just walked out, and it did not affect me at all. I laid a complaint with his employer who did nothing about it so I escalated it to the Australian Human Rights Commission. They advised that I had a valid complaint and that they were going to investigate the incident.

I no longer take crap from anyone regarding my impairment and nor should I. Although I have to say, I am now more inclined to use either my telephone app or sign language.

Depression

Time passed, so quickly I might add, but I had some really, really bad days. Think of the worst day you have ever had and multiple it by 1000.

Not long ago I had a very bad case of depression that lasted a lot longer than before. The only thing that kept me from acting on the negative thoughts that I had, was my wife and the thought of what it would do to her.

My neighbour of twenty-plus years lost her husband to the big 'C' seven months ago, so when I am at home by myself, I go check on her to make sure that she is okay. This serves two purposes: I make sure she is okay and that she knows that someone cares about her and it distracts me long enough to get over the thoughts or depressive mood I am having.

I spoke to my psychologist about it and she said with what I have been through and lost, I should expect to have bad days for some time. She said that I was entitled to them. The key is how you deal with them.

We talked about several strategies on how to deal with those bad days, but ideally, we want to work on reducing both the frequency and duration of those bad days.

One solution which works for me is exercise and this works for me in several ways. It releases the endorphins that make me feel better.

My assistance dog needs exercising and continual training and I want to start my fundraising project.

Exercise

So, let's talk about exercise. One day I looked in the mirror, and other than being ugly, I had lots of loose skin. My bottom looked like an old elephant with heaps of loose saggy skin. I suppose that happens when you were 110 kilograms when this journey started and now I'm at 67 kilograms, the lightest I've ever been.

A friend of my wife recommended to us a Physical Training Instructor that he uses. She is very reasonably priced, very experienced and she comes to you.

So that was my starting point. I now see her twice a week, every week for the last five months and we do cross-fit. I have to say that with putting on 8 kilograms in weight and the exercise, I don't look that bad now, other than being ugly and no one can help me with that.

My blood pressure has come down, my resting heart rate has also come down and I get more unaided sleep. How do I know that? Well I have a Fitbit watch and it helps track everything from food, exercise, heart rate, sleep and drink intake, just to mention some of the benefits.

In addition to the cross-fit I also have a structured exercise program four days a week. Over the next nine months I intend to go from a couch potato to running in excess of twenty-five kilometres per week.

PERTH HEAD AND NECK CANCER SUPPORT

Well I have taken what has happened with a passion. Employment is not possible, so I had to come up with something else to keep me occupied. I have a strong desire to help other people who are about to, are currently or have dealt with head and neck cancer.

There is a lack of head and neck cancer support in Western Australia. A wise person once said to me, if you see a problem and nobody is doing anything about it, then fix it yourself. Problem: there is no support group in Western Australia for head and neck cancer.

Solution — I started the Perth Head and Neck Cancer Support Group with the goal of:

1. Helping other people who are about to start dealing with, currently dealing with or who have dealt with head and neck cancer.

2. Highlight and increase awareness of head and neck cancer, in Western Australia.

3. Provide resources to those researching head and neck cancer.

I made a Facebook page, and in the matter of two hours

I had thirteen supporters. I had discussions with Fiona Stanley Hospital, and they are very keen for me to hold the meetings at the hospital.

This will enable me to advertise the support group at the hospital and Cancer Council of WA.

From the small beginnings great things happen.

The other thing is to increase the awareness, education and research for Head & Neck Cancer in Western Australia. So, I have started the Western Australian Head & Neck Cancer Support Foundation. I am currently building this up so that we can help the Support Group, patients and carers and provide money for research.

Getting back to my exercise goal? The second idea I had was huge and it just reinforced in some people that I really am crazy. I am currently in the process of organising a 1,550-kilometre marathon relay charity run, from the Western Australian/South Australian border to Fiona Stanley Hospital.

Now my goal is to be one of those five runners and it is proposed that we each do twenty kilometres each per day, with one runner running at a time.

Besides sponsorship it is intended that money will also be raised along the route. I have a goal of raising at least $350,000 for Western Australian Head and Neck Cancer Support Foundation between sponsorships and donations.

I am in the process of getting promotional material done up, sponsors and of course the all-important task of recruiting four more runners. Now if I can't get four more runners, simple I'll do it myself and it takes a little longer that's all.

Employment

I had an employment survey conducted and had them look at two things. The first - would a law firm employ a lawyer with severe speech impairment, especially one that wanted to specialise in Safety, Workers Compensation and Industrial Law.

The second was looking at the possibility of being employed as a safety professional.

The report came back not in a positive manner, which I was sort of expecting. It seems that I had more chances of winning first division lotto, five consecutive times in a row.

So employment for what I was trained to do was not possible and I have withdrawn from university.

Assistance Dog

In my Final Rules chapter (at the back) I say get a dog. Well with the choking issues that I have had and the fact that I collapsed twice, I got myself a German Shepherd. In my case, I got an 18-months old male.

I have two trainers that are helping me. The first one is helping with obedience training and with learning how to control my dog with sign language.

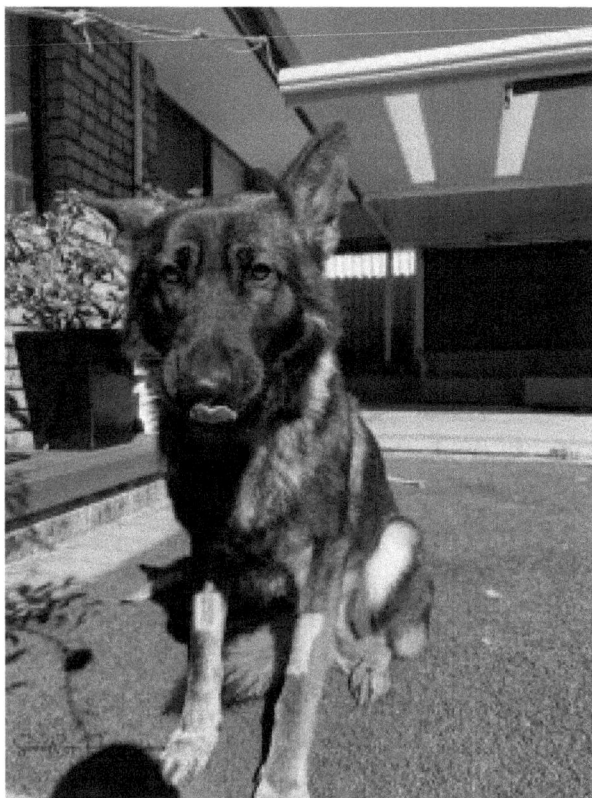

The second trainer is training my dog in three assistance tasks. These are:

1. Comfort me when I am depressed, and believe me, he knows when I am down.

2. To press my man down alarm. This is an alarm that most older people get when they live alone, fall and cannot ring for help, they push the button for help. In my case it sends a text message to eight people, then commences to ring those eight people in turn. When it is answered the device becomes a two-way telephone, so the person can talk to me.

3. The third and final task is to jump on my chest (or back if face down) and force air out of my lungs. Doctors tell me that this will be enough to lodge free the obstruction and allow me to breathe.

Besides the training, the dog also forces me to exercise.

Latest Cancer Results

So it was that time of year again, March. PET scan time and a case of *scanxiety* and boy, it is always a concern, and this time it was no exception. The results were once again cancer free. Getting closer to the five-year mark.

FINAL RULES

→ When you're in a tough situation, break it down into manageable steps. Literally, if need be. You will be able to focus on exactly what you need to be doing at that very moment and prevent being overwhelmed by the overall task.

→ Consistency of effort over an extended period of time will yield results. Guaranteed.

→ Be persistent and dogged in your determination to get better and survive. Mental toughness is like a muscle — the more you work at it, the stronger it becomes.

→ Remember to breathe! Deep, rhythmic and consistent breathing will allow you to handle stress better and remain calm, focused and in control.

→   Control what you can.

→   Let go of what you can't and <u>ask</u> for help.

→   Research exactly what you're getting into, what you need to survive and function.

→   Be prepared. I cannot stress this enough. Be prepared.

→   Realise when you may be over your head and out of your depth, then rely on the medical practitioners and nurses to get you through this, that's their profession and they are good at it.

→   Learn from your mistakes. If something didn't work, think of another way.

→   Be willing to constantly improve your mindset and do little things for yourself.

→   Keep your head up and stay positive.

→   Live for the present and not the past, nor too far into the future.

→   Get a dog. A dog will give you unconditional friendship and love, especially when you are alone. It will also mean that you have to take it for a walk and exercise will only assist in your recovery. Ask your medical practitioner before going for a walk first.

➜ **This is survivable and you can and will survive. I have and if I can, <u>you</u> can.**

FINAL CHAPTER

Someone asked me two questions. The first one was, what had I learned from all of this and the second one was why I took the time and trouble to write this booklet and then the Epilogue.

What have I learnt from all of this and what am I still learning each day?

→ Some people just don't get what a cancer sufferer goes through.

→ Family is very important. They can be your only true friends even though you may not know it.

→ Friendship can't be taken for granted. Love the friends that stick with you, as they are precious.

→ Friends will leave you as they are scared for themselves.

→ Being and doing are different, but are linked, neither exists without the other.

→ One of the biggest lessons I have learnt, is to enjoy my own company.

→ Once you come out the other side of this journey, it is a new beginning.

→ Work out what you can control and don't worry about the rest.

→ Set realistic goals and work out the strategies to achieve them.

→ The only person who has been on this complete journey is me and me alone. I am the one person who must steer this vessel and confront the various situations, both physical and mental along with emotional.

→ Focus on what you want and not want you don't want.

→ Focus on getting well and remaining well. Be selfish about succeeding.

→ Relax and take time out for yourself.

→ The human body can take a lot of punishment and endure a lot of pain. It is the mind that has a problem keeping up.

→ Learn to look after yourself.

→ Finding balance in your life is important. You must learn to have your physical, mental and emotional selves in balance.

→ Remember what you have been through and don't let anyone take that away from you.

→ One of the problems that I am having at the moment is learning how to value yourself. I often wonder what value I am both to myself and my wife. My wife tells me that I am very valuable and have a lot to offer to both her and society.

→ The mind is a powerful tool, use all the tools you have on this journey.

→ Don't take life for granted.

The reason I wrote this was for two reasons. First, because at the time, I felt there was a lack of information around from someone who had actually lived and dealt with head and neck cancer.

Second, is so that I could remember what I have been through and the lessons I learnt, not only about myself, but head and neck cancer; something that I knew nothing about before all of this, yet it has had such a huge impact on me and society.

I actually lived this ordeal and most importantly, did NOT give up. I survived. I hope this helps just one person who has to go through what I went through so that they can also become a 12%er, like me.

I also intend to be a 71%er (up from 63% in 2018), and survive in five years' time, but time will tell.

With modern medical advances, not only has the survival rate increased in the last two years, but so has the incidence rate.

In 2017, the Western Australian incidence rate for head and neck cancer was 584 people. Of these 584 unfortunately 115 died.

In 2019, there were 5,212 new cases of head and neck cancer diagnosed in Australia and this accounts for 3.4% of all cancers diagnosed.

That number is expected to increase in 2020. In 2019, it was estimated that there are 17,000 people living with head and neck cancer in Australia.

Survivors of cancer have unique and ongoing healthcare needs, with many facing physical, psychological and financial challenges upon diagnosis, during and after their treatment. Patient expectations are changing with an increasing focus on their experience of cancer control, including the provision of holistic support and the best possible quality of life.

Please donate to head and neck cancer research and support: **www.waheadandneckcancer.org.au**

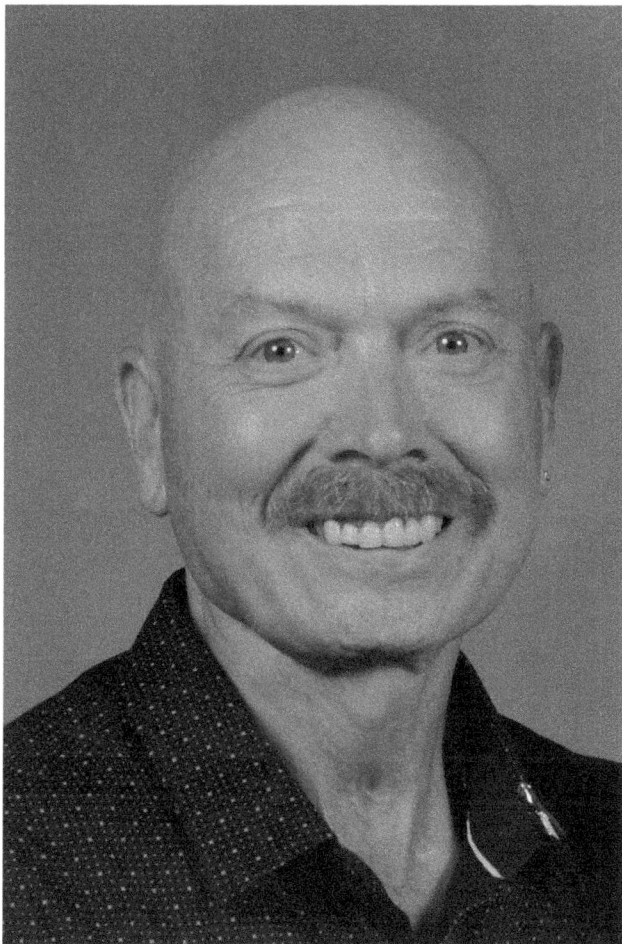

Me today.